STROKE:

A Nurse's Guide to Caring for the Patient

Jillian Riske, MSN, RN-BC, PCCN
Kate Culver, MSN, RN, PCCN

Cover created by Katie Swaim Design

Ordering Information
Quantity sales: Special discounts are available on quantity purchases by corporations, associations, and others. For details, contact the publisher at the above email address.

Printed in the United States of America.

ISBN 13: 978-0-9981114-0-7
ISBN 10: 0-9981114-0-6

Disclaimer
The information provided herein is stated to be truthful and consistent, in that any liability, in terms of inattention or otherwise, by any usage or abuse of any policies, processes, or directions contained within is the solitary and utter responsibility of the recipient reader. Under no circumstances will any legal responsibility or blame be held against the publisher for any reparation, damages, or monetary loss due to the information herein, either directly or indirectly.

The information herein is offered for informational purposes solely, and is universal as so. The presentation of the information is without contract or any type of guarantee assurance.

The trademarks that are used are without any consent, and the publication of the trademark is without permission or backing by the trademark owner. All trademarks and brands within this book are for clarifying purposes only and are owned by the owners themselves, not affiliated with this document.

CONTENTS

ABOUT THE AUTHORS

JILLIAN RISKE, MSN, RN-BC, PCCN, completed her bachelor's of science degree in nursing from the University of Texas at Austin and her master's degree in nursing administration at the University of Texas at Arlington. Jillian has been working in health care for over ten years. She started as a patient care and monitor technician while in nursing school. After school, she transitioned to her role as a critical care nurse where she found a passion for cardiac and neuro patients. She has served in various roles that include bedside nurse, preceptor, charge nurse, and supervisor. Jillian has also taught classes on critical care and cardiac topics.

Early in her career, Jillian completed a specialty nurse fellowship through the hospital where she is employed. Through this fellowship, she implemented the use of a sepsis-screening tool that led to earlier detection of sepsis in patients. She went on to present her findings in a poster presentation at the American Association of Critical Care Nurses National Conference in Washington, D.C. Through her work in the fellowship, she was recognized with a professional contribution award.

Jillian is a member of the American Association of Critical Care nurses and a past member of Sigma Theta Tau. She holds various certifications in her specialty, including progressive care and board certification.

Jillian resides in Austin, Texas, where she and her husband raise their two young boys. She continues to enjoy bedside nursing and has plans to continue writing books to help nurses better understand how to care for their patients.

Publication: Abstract for National Teaching Institute Creative Solutions poster published in *Critical Care Nurse Journal:* Riske, J. & Butz, M. (2010). CS42 A New Screening Strategy Detects Sepsis and Prevents Septic Shock. *Crit Care Nurse,* 30.

KATE CULVER, MSN, RN, PCCN, has been in health care for nearly a decade. While attending Nursing School at the University of Oklahoma, she began working as a patient care technician in a hospital. After graduating with her bachelor's of science in nursing in 2008, she moved to Austin, Texas, where she began working as a graduate nurse for a well-known hospital organization in the cardiac and intermediate care setting. During her five years spent on that unit as a staff nurse, she gained experience in the specialty through a fellowship program, precepting new hires, and charge nursing. Through these experiences and the support of nursing leadership, Kate was able to obtain her progressive care nursing certification.

Eventually, Kate returned to school to obtain her master's of science in nursing administration degree and teaching certificate from the University of Texas at Arlington. After graduating in 2012, she gained experience as a nurse educator in the critical care, orthopedic, and neuroscience specialties. During that time, she was given the opportunity to create simulation scenarios for the hospital partnership's new hire nurses, conduct lectures on critical care and stroke related topics, validate competencies in nursing skills, and become certified in teaching both basic and advanced cardiac life support classes. This is when her love for teaching was fostered and why she wants to continue contributing to the nursing profession through education. Kate currently works as a nurse manager in the acute care setting on units that primarily care for the Neuroscience and Orthopedic patient population.

Kate lives in Austin with her husband, cat, dog, and growing family. They love taking full advantage of outdoor activities, hike and bike trails and exceptional cuisine Austin has to offer.

INTRODUCTION

Hello,

We would like to thank you for buying our book, *Stroke: A Nurses' Guide to Caring for the Patient.*

We have spent a combined 20 years working in many different nursing disciplines. During this time, we have trained hundreds of nurses. We have taken the knowledge and stories we have shared with them and written a book to share with all nurses. We hope that this book provides a simple and easy-to-understand guide to caring for your patients.

The intended audience for this book is nursing students, graduate nurses, and nurses who are new to caring for stroke patients. The information is explained in a simplified and easy-to-understand manner.

Please visit our website to find out more information about Nurseology and the products we provide. And please feel free to provide feedback or suggestions to info@nurseology.com.

Enjoy!

Jill and Kate

1
ANATOMY AND PHYSIOLOGY

What is a stroke? As a nurse, you already have an idea of what a stroke is. But how is it defined? A stroke is an acute vascular event that affects the brain and involves neurological changes as a result of an interruption of blood supply to one or more parts of the brain. This can be caused by a reduction or a complete absence of blood flow to an area of the brain. This absence in blood flow damages the tissue surrounding the area. The amount of time the area has been without blood determines the amount of damage that will be caused.

Stroke is one of the top leading causes of death in the United States. Strokes are responsible for half of all neuro-related hospitalizations and are the primary cause of long-term disability in adults.

Understanding the brain, how it works, and how it affects what we do every day is an important part of caring for someone who has had a stroke. The brain is an extremely complex organ, as you already know, and people often find it to be the most intimidating to learn about. Let's start with the brain's anatomy. (See Figure 1.)

Parts of the Brain

- *Frontal lobe*: Our emotional headquarters and home to our personality
- *Parietal lobe*: Can be separated into 2 regions of function: sensation and perception
- *Occipital lobe*: Home of our visual perception system
- *Temporal lobe*: Responsible for object categorization, memories, and emotions
- *Cerebellum*: Involved in voluntary motor movements, balance, equilibrium, and muscle movement
- *Brain stem*: Responsible for vital functions, digestion, and sleep

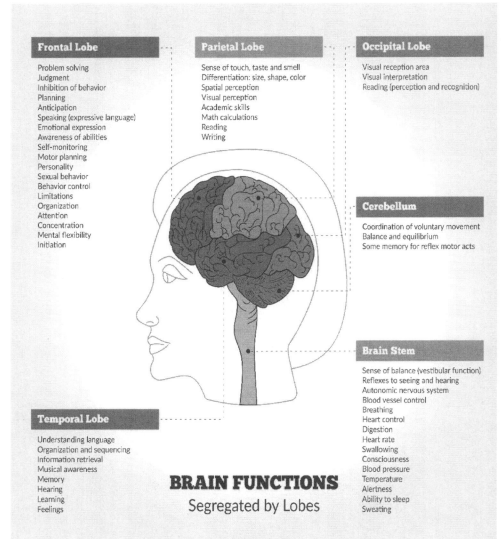

Frontal Lobe

Problem solving
Judgment
Inhibition of behavior
Planning
Anticipation
Speaking (expressive language)
Emotional expression
Awareness of abilities
Self-monitoring
Motor planning
Personality
Sexual behavior
Behavior control
Limitations
Organization
Attention
Concentration
Mental flexibility
Initiation

Parietal Lobe

Sense of touch, taste and smell
Differentiation: size, shape, color
Spatial perception
Visual perception
Academic skills
Math calculations
Reading
Writing

Occipital Lobe

Visual reception area
Visual interpretation
Reading (perception and recognition)

Cerebellum

Coordination of voluntary movement
Balance and equilibrium
Some memory for reflex motor acts

Brain Stem

Sense of balance (vestibular function)
Reflexes to seeing and hearing
Autonomic nervous system
Blood vessel control
Breathing
Heart control
Digestion
Heart rate
Swallowing
Consciousness
Blood pressure
Temperature
Alertness
Ability to sleep
Sweating

Temporal Lobe

Understanding language
Organization and sequencing
Information retrieval
Musical awareness
Memory
Hearing
Learning
Feelings

BRAIN FUNCTIONS

Segregated by Lobes

FIGURE 1: BRAIN FUNCTIONS

10

Blood Supply

Two major sets of arteries supply blood to the brain:

1. *Internal carotid arteries*: Supply the front, or anterior, portion of the brain. This also includes the frontal, temporal, and parietal lobes as well as the basal ganglia.
2. *Vertebral arteries*: Housed in the cervical vertebral column and supply blood to the back, or posterior, portion of the brain. This includes the temporal and occipital lobes, cerebellum, brain stem, thalamus, and hypothalamus.

Branching off those are the anterior, middle, and posterior cerebral arteries. (See Figure 2.)

- *Anterior cerebral artery*: Extends upward and forward from the internal carotid artery. It supplies the frontal lobe, the parts of the brain that control logical thought, personality, and voluntary movement primarily in the lower limbs.
- *Middle cerebral artery*: Often referred to as the MCA, this artery is the most common area for occlusive strokes and is the largest branch off the internal carotid artery. It supplies blood to the frontal, temporal, and parietal lobes, including the primary motor and sensory areas of the face, throat, hands, upper limbs, and areas of speech for the dominant hemisphere. The MCA also feeds the basal ganglia and the internal capsule.
- *Posterior cerebral artery*: The posterior cerebral artery typically stems from the basilar artery. It is responsible for supplying the temporal and occipital lobes. When infarction occurs in this vessel, it is usually secondary to embolism from lower portions of the vertebral basilar system or heart.

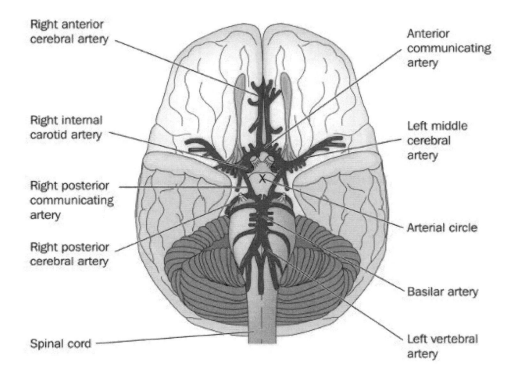

Right anterior cerebral artery

Anterior communicating artery

Right internal carotid artery

Left middle cerebral artery

Right posterior communicating artery

Right posterior cerebral artery

Arterial circle

Basilar artery

Spinal cord

Left vertebral artery

FIGURE 2: CIRCLE OF WILLIS

In chapter 2, we talk more about the symptoms you might see when each of these lobes and vessels has been affected by a stroke.

Now that you have an understanding of the basic anatomy of the brain, let's discuss what causes strokes and the different types of strokes a person can have.

Risk Factors

Some risk factors a person can change (modifiable), and some cannot be changed (nonmodifiable). These risk factors are extremely important to discuss with a patient when providing patient education. It is also important to differentiate between what is modifiable and what is not and to make sure your patient or the patient's family understands this when he is discharged from the hospital.

Modifiable Risk Factors

- Atrial fibrillation
- Coronary artery disease
- Diabetes
- Heart disease
- Hypertension
- High cholesterol
- Illicit drug use (e.g., cocaine)
- Obesity
- Sedentary lifestyle
- Smoking and/or alcohol intake

Nonmodifiable Risk Factors

- Age
- Family history of brain or heart vessel disease
- Gender
- Previous stroke/TIA
- Race and ethnicity

Transient Ischemic Attack (TIA)

Transient ischemic attacks, also known as TIAs, are often referred to as "ministrokes." The symptoms typically resolve within 24 hours. A TIA occurs when a clot occludes a vessel temporarily. However, if someone has a TIA, she is significantly more likely to have a stroke, so this is another invaluable point of education for patients and families.

TIAs do not cause an infarct in the brain, but you want to treat these patients as if they have had an actual stroke. This is simply to be extra cautious. You always want to be this way when taking care of patients. If there is a suspected TIA, but the patient has actually had a small stroke, you want to be sure you have completed all the appropriate tests, have given the correct medications, and have taken all the necessary precautions for these patients while under your care.

Let's take a closer look at strokes.

So, what are the different types of strokes a person can have? There are 2 major types of stroke: ischemic and hemorrhagic. Ischemic strokes make up a little more than 85% of all strokes.

Ischemic Stroke

- *Thrombus*: Formed in local vessel
- *Embolus*: Formed elsewhere and travelled to brain
- *Lacunar infarct*: Occurs in a penetrating artery that supplies deeper parts of the brain
- *Hypoperfusion*: Decreased blood flow to the brain

Ischemic strokes have 2 areas of injury:

1. *Core ischemic area*: This area is closest to the blockage of blood flow. It has very poor to no perfusion that may result in necrosis of neurons.
2. *Penumbra:* This is the area around the core ischemia where there is some ischemia, but neurons may still be viable. This area is where reperfusion therapies are most likely to be successful in restoring neurons.

Hemorrhagic Stroke

This type of stroke causes the patient to complain of a severe headache. Patients often describe it as the "worst headache of my life." It is caused by leakage of blood from a vessel into the brain or parts surrounding the brain.

Intracerebral Hemorrhage (ICH)

- Bleeding directly into the brain
- Result of a ruptured vessel

- Commonly caused by coagulation disorders, anticoagulant medications, trauma, rupture of aneurysms, vascular malformations, and tumors
- Gathering of blood in the area can occur over minutes to hours

Subarachnoid Hemorrhage (SAH)
- Leaking of blood into cerebrospinal fluid (CSF)
- Commonly caused by aneurysm rupture or bleeding of arteriovenous malformations (AVM) but may also be the result of illicit drug use or trauma

What is an aneurysm? An aneurysm is a weakened area of the vessel wall that may be congenital or acquired. Aneurysms vary in type and size, but all present as a terrible headache when ruptured or leaking.

What is an arteriovenous malformation? Often referred to by its acronym, an AVM is a mass of arteries and veins that appear to be tangled with one another.

2
ASSESSMENT

The nursing assessment is an important tool for tailoring the care of a stroke patient. If you have a general understanding of the type of stroke, where it occurred, and which areas of the brain were affected, you will know what deficits to expect and what specific safety precautions you should take when caring for your patient.

Let's talk about what deficits you can expect based on which side of the brain, the area, and which vessel was affected by the stroke. Remember, every stroke patient is different and will likely not present with the same deficits as other stroke patients you care for, which is why a thorough neurological assessment is so crucial. Similar to your nursing head-to-toe assessment, you can also complete your neurological assessments starting at the head and making your way down to your patient's legs and feet.

Common Stroke Symptoms
- Numbness, tingling, or weakness in the face, arms, or legs
- Confusion, trouble speaking or understanding
- Vision loss or difficulty seeing things
- Difficulty walking
- Severe headache

Effects of a Left Brain Versus Right Brain Injury
Left Brain
- Detailed information analysis
- Intellectual ability
- Slow and cautious behavior
- Right-sided paralysis and weakness
- Memory for spoken or written messages

Right Brain
- Left-sided weakness or paralysis
- Body position
- Impulsive behavior
- Left visual field deficit
- Spatial and perceptual field deficits
- Vague emotional response
- Increased distractibility

Signs Based on the Area of the Brain Affected by Stroke
Frontal Lobe
- Loss of simple body movement (paralysis)
- Loss of flexibility in thinking
- Persistence on a single thought
- Inability to focus on a task
- Mood changes
- Changes in social behavior
- Changes in personality
- Difficulty with problem solving
- Inability to express language (also called Broca's aphasia)

Keep in mind that these frontal lobe deficits can often look like dementia or Parkinson's disease. Be sure that you can differentiate between stroke symptoms and, most important, the presentation of a new stroke versus underlying neurological diseases.

Parietal Lobe
- Lack of ability to focus on more than 1 object at a time
- Inability to name objects (known as anomia)
- Problems with reading (known as alexia)
- Difficulty drawing objects and with math (known as dyscalculia)
- Inability to locate words for writing (known as agraphia)
- Difficulty with hand–eye coordination

Occipital Lobe
- Visual deficits
- Problems locating objects, distinguishing colors, recognizing drawn objects, reading, and writing
- Possible hallucinations
- Inability to recognize the movement of objects (known as agnosia)

Temporal Lobe
- Difficulty with auditory and visual input and perception
- Inability to understand spoken word
- Memory loss
- Increase or decrease in sexual behavior
- Increased aggressive behavior
- Persistent talking (right temporal lobe damage)

Cerebellum
- Unable to coordinate fine motor movement
- Inability to walk
- Tremors
- Difficulty grabbing objects
- Vertigo
- Slow movement
- Slurred speech

Brain Stem
- Difficulty swallowing (known as dysphagia)
- Decreased respiratory function
- Difficulty organizing thoughts and perception of surroundings
- Problems with balance and coordination (known as ataxia)
- Involuntary eye movement (known as nystagmus)
- Sleep disturbances, such as apnea and insomnia
- Dizziness and nausea from vertigo

Components of the Neurological Assessment

When completing a head-to-toe neurological assessment, assess both the right and the left sides of the patient. We encourage you to review your neurological assessment finding with the oncoming shift to clarify that you are both seeing the same thing. This will minimize any confusion if you have left for the day and the oncoming nurses assess the pupils to be a different size, or the left leg is weaker to them than what you have documented.

Mental Status

The patient's mental status and level of consciousness provide very important information about neurological function. This is an opportunity to ask the patient about his name, date, what city he is in, and who the president is. This gives you an idea of his orientation. Be patient, and give him time to answer these questions.

The Glasgow coma scale will also give you a quantifiable level of mental status.

- *Level of consciousness*: Is the patient alert, awake; arouses to voice, touch, or painful stimuli?
- *Orientation*: Is the patient oriented to person, place, time, and situation?
- *Respiratory pattern*: Is the patient breathing at a normal rate and rhythm? Too fast or too slow?
- *Pupils*: How do pupils respond to light? Move a penlight from the lateral side of the patient's face to the front, and examine the pupils. How big are they? How do they react to the light?
- *Clarity of speech*: Do you notice any slurring? Or is the speech clear?
- *Language*: Is what the patient saying appropriate? Is the patient nonverbal?

Cranial Nerves

- Olfactory: smell (not usually tested)
- Optic: visual acuity
- Oculomotor: opening of eyes, all eye movement
- Trochlear: downward and medial eye movement
- Trigeminal: chewing movements, face sensation
- Abducens: lateral eye movement

- Facial: eyelid closing, facial muscle movement
- Auditory: hearing and ability to balance
- Glossopharyngeal: taste (not usually tested)
- Vagus: uvula and swallowing
- Accessory: shoulder shrug
- Hypoglossal: tongue movement

Motor Assessment

Motor assessment techniques test muscle innervation by the spinal nerves. It is important to determine if any weakness is present and to assess muscle tone.

Evaluation of arm drift is a sensitive test for weakness in the upper extremities. Instruct the patient to extend her arms straight out, with palms up and eyes closed. If the patient is experiencing some weakness, you will see these limbs drift downward. Ask the patient to squeeze your hands to determine her level of strength as well. Moving to the lower limbs, ask the patient to attempt plantar flexion and dorsiflexion against the force of your hands.

Observe and test muscles for flaccidity, spasticity, or rigidity. Look for any muscle atrophy while you are examining the muscles.

Sensory Examination

The basic sensory examination in nursing consists primarily of pain and light touch. The location of tingling, burning, or numbness will identify which dermatome has been affected by the stroke. Test the affected and adjacent dermatomes bilaterally with a pin prick and light touch to determine whether any sensory loss has occurred.

Reflexes

Perform the Babinski reflex by holding the patient's foot with one hand and stroking the lateral aspect of the sole from the heel toward the ball of the foot with a pointed object, such as a pen or tongue depressor. A positive Babinski sign is characterized by flexion and a fanning of the toes, which indicates a problem with the central nervous system.

Safety Assessment

- Airway
- Fall risk (impulsive, confused)
- Bleeding risk (anticoagulants, bleeding disorder)
- Tendency to pull at drains, tubes, or IV access
- Dysphagia

You may notice that some of these deficits overlap at different areas of the brain, making your assessment more challenging. Fine-tuning this skill will make you that much more aware of how to care for your stroke patient. As we mentioned before, not all symptoms associated with one area of the brain will present themselves while you are assessing your patient. Often times, some symptoms of 2 or more areas may be present. Use your thorough neurological assessment skills to determine which areas of the brain might be involved in your patient's stroke and use that to understand why the patient might behave the way he does, what safety precautions you need to use, and how to teach the patient's family more about what they might experience from the patient as well.

Nothing replaces a thorough head-to-toe neurological examination. However, you can use several assessment tools for a quick assessment before the official neurological assessment takes place.

One tool, known as the Cincinnati Prehospital Stroke Scale, is commonly used in the community and for patient education. It utilizes the acronym FAST to quickly detect the signs and symptoms of a stroke.

F–Face **A**–Arm **S**–Speech **T**–Time

Secondly, the National Institutes of Health certifies nurses in completing the NIH Stroke Scale.

NIH Stroke Scale

The National Institutes for Health Stroke Scale (NIHSS) is a standardized stroke severity scale used to describe neurological deficits in acute stroke patients. It allows health care professionals to quickly quantify their clinical exam and determine whether the patient's neurological status is improving or declining.

The NIHSS employs an 11-item scoring system. The maximum score possible is 42; the minimum score is zero. The stroke scale tests the following:
- Level of consciousness
- Best gaze
- Visual field testing
- Facial paresis
- Arm and leg motor function
- Limb ataxia
- Sensory
  - Best language\dysarthria

- Extinction and inattention

When conducting the NIHSS, the most reproducible response is generally the first response, and that is what you should use for your score.
- Do not coach patient unless specified.
- Give the patient a score based on what you actually see the patient do, not what you think the patient can do.
- The higher a patient's score, the greater the patient has been affected by the stroke.
    - > 25: very severe neurological impairment
    - 15–24: severe impairment
    - 5–14: moderately severe impairment
    - < 5: mild impairment
- The initial NIHSS is a probable indicator of the patient's discharge disposition.
- A 2-point, or greater, increase on the NIHSS administered serially indicates stroke progression. Call the doctor when this is noted unless otherwise ordered.
- An NIHSS should also be completed on discharge and compared with the score given on admission.

3
ORDERS

This chapter is divided into orders you will receive in the emergency department, general stroke admission orders, and then specific orders for hemorrhagic and ischemic strokes. We have included rationale so that you can better understand why you may receive these types of orders.

When a patient is brought into the emergency room with stroke-like symptoms, the most important things you can do as the nurse is to assist getting the patient to the CT scanner as quickly as possible and to obtain a good history. The CT scan will determine the type of stroke the patient is having and the type of treatment the patient will require. A detailed history is important to find out when the patient was "last known well." This term is a common phrase used when determining the last time a patient was seen without symptoms. Knowing this provides a critical timeline to determine the appropriate treatment.

Emergency Department Orders
- Establish IV access.
- Check vital signs every 15 minutes.
- Maintain continuous cardiac and oxygen-saturation monitoring.
- Keep O_2 > 92%.
- Activity: bedrest.
- Make neuro checks every 15 minutes.

- Assess for any worsening or improvement of symptoms. Notify the physician immediately if symptoms worsen.

NPO Until Swallow Screen Is Completed

The patient may have a diminished swallow after a stroke. You can perform a preliminary swallow screen if your hospital policy allows. To do this, allow the patient to drink small amounts of water (5 ml, 15 ml, and a glass of water). Stop if the patient coughs or has trouble swallowing. If the patient is too sleepy or unable to participate, stop the swallow screen, make the patient NPO, and request a speech therapist to perform a swallow screen.

Noncontrast Computed Tomography Scan

This head scan is done in the radiology department and takes about 5 minutes. It should be obtained as quickly as possible.

EKG

An EKG may be obtained to determine if the patient is in atrial fibrillation. This type of rhythm can cause blood clots in the heart that can travel to the brain and trigger an ischemic stroke. Also, it is important to rule out any cardiac events, such as a myocardial infarction.

Labs

- Complete blood count (CBC)
- Comprehensive metabolic panel (CMP or comp)
- PT/PTT
- Cardiac enzymes
- Lipid panel
- Blood glucose level

27

- HgA1C

All of these are standard labs ordered to establish a baseline and look for any abnormal values that may be contributing to the cause of the presenting problem.

A PT/PTT looks at how thin the blood is. It is important to know the PT/PTT if the patient is having a hemorrhagic stroke. This is especially important to know for patients who are on blood thinners. It may be necessary to give reversal agents if the patient has a high PT/PTT.

If tPA is given, then a baseline CBC and PT/PTT is important to have because tPA can cause bleeding.

It is important to rule hypoglycemia out as a cause of the presenting symptoms because low blood glucose levels can mimic stroke symptoms.

tPA
See chapter 6, "Critical Care and Interventions," for details on tPA administration.

General Stroke Orders
Some patients may require admission to ICU or other closely monitored units, depending on the severity of their stroke. Often times these patients may need IV medications or frequent neuro checks.

Activity Level
The activity level ordered will depend on the severity of the stroke.

Neuro Checks

Assess for any worsening or improvement of symptoms. Notify the physician immediately if symptoms worsen.

Vital Signs

It is common for patients who have had a stroke to have elevated blood pressure. With ischemic strokes, doctors may allow the blood pressure to elevate. This is called permissive hypertension. The increase in blood pressure can help perfuse the area of the brain that is infarcted. You may see orders to treat blood pressures only greater than 220/110. (This is OK. We know it doesn't seem right.)

For patients who have had hemorrhagic strokes, the blood pressure control is much tighter. Systolic blood pressure should be kept < 160. Poor blood pressure control could result in further bleeding in the brain.

It is common for stroke patients to have a slightly elevated temperature. This is caused by the brain's reaction to the stroke, not an infectious process. You may see tighter parameters to treat the fever > 99.6°F (37.6°C).

Swallow Screen

The swallow screen may have already been completed in the emergency department, but if it hasn't, you may perform one at the bedside.

Speech Therapy

Speech therapy may be ordered to assist the patient with swallowing, determining the best modified diet, cognition, and/or communication.

Diet

Speech therapy will help guide the doctors and nurses on what type of diet is appropriate. The food options include regular, diced, ground, and pureed. The drink options include thin, honey thick, and nectar thick. You can use a thickener to make any beverage the appropriate consistency.

Some patients are not safe to swallow any food or liquid. These patients may have a feeding tube placed in their nose. They may be on a continuous feeding pump of liquid nutrition through their feeding tube. Consult your dietician to help the doctor determine the appropriate nutritional supplement the patient should receive.

Physical and Occupational Therapy

Often times after a stroke, patients have weakness on one side of their body. Physical therapy can help these patients regain some or all of their strength through exercises. Occupational therapy will assist the patient in the same manner but focus more on helping the patients to resume and/or modify their activities of daily living so that they may maintain their independence.

Blood Glucose Checks

Diabetic patients are at higher risk for stroke. It is important to monitor and maintain these patients' blood sugar. NPO patients should be checked every 6 hours. Patients who are eating should be checked AC/HS. Sliding-scale insulin should be ordered for diabetic patients.

Diagnostic Tests

- *Magnetic resonance imaging (MRI)*: a detailed scan of the brain that is useful to assess areas of ischemia, hemorrhage, and infarction
- *MR angiography (MRA)*: a detailed scan that looks at the blood flow in the brain. It may show narrowing or blockage of the arteries in the neck and/or brain, and the presence of an aneurysm.
- *Transcranial doppler (TCD)*: an ultrasound that looks at cerebral blood flow (It is useful for detecting the presence of vasospasms in the brain.)
- *Carotid ultrasound*: an ultrasound used to assess blood flow through the carotid arteries (The carotid ultrasound will show the presence of plaque buildup that can occlude blood flow to the brain.)
- *CT angio head and neck*: Similar to an MRA, a CT angio looks at the blood flow in the brain. It may be used to assess for narrowing of the vessels in the brain or to search for the presence of an aneurysm.
- *Electroencephalogram (EEG)*: examines the brains electrical activity (Useful in determining the presence of seizure activity. The patient must be able to lie still for 1 to 2 hours while the test is conducted.)
- *Echocardiogram (echo)*: a motion picture of the heart's blood flow used to look for the source of emboli

Ischemic Stroke Orders
Telemetry
Continuous cardiac monitoring may be ordered to watch for the presence of arrhythmias that caused the ischemic stroke—more specifically, atrial fibrillation.

- *Blood pressure management*: Treat if BP is greater than 220/110.
  - Clonidine: usually ordered as PO PRN
  - Labetalol: usually ordered as IV PRN
- *Antithrombotics*: Reduce the formation of clots and help to reduce stroke reoccurrence.
  - Aggrenox, Plavix, aspirin (may use rectally while NPO)
- *IV fluids*: May be necessary while NPO. IV fluids can be useful in improving cerebral blood flow in dehydrated patients.

Hemorrhagic Stroke Orders
Consult Neurosurgeon
Patients with hemorrhagic strokes may be candidates for neurosurgical interventions. (See chapter 6, "Critical Care and Interventions," for more details.)

Blood Pressure Management
Keep SBP < 160.

- Labetalol: usually available as IV PRN
- Apresoline: usually available as IV or PO PRN
- Nicardipine: given as an IV titrating drip; typically ordered in critical-care areas where the patient can be closely monitored

Vasospasms

The doctor may order daily transcranial dopplers (TCD) to look for vasospasms.

- Nimodipine: Calcium channel blocker that helps prevent occurrence of vasospasms after subarachnoid hemorrhage. ***Caution: May cause hypotension.***

Management of Swelling

- Dexamethasone: steroid that reduces swelling and antiinflammatory response
- Mannitol: diuretic that reduces cerebral edema (It is important to check serum osmolality and a basic metabolic panel every 12 hours while on mannitol. Do not give if serum osmolality is > 320. This would indicate that too much fluid is being taken out.)

Pain Management

Administering pain medication to patients who have had strokes can be challenging because the effects of opioid narcotics can mimic worsening stroke symptoms. It is best to try to give medications that are least sedating. If narcotics must be given, fentanyl is an ideal medication because of its short half-life. Some nursing units may not be able to administer this medication.

4
COMPLICATIONS

Brain swelling (cerebral edema or herniation) is the increase of fluid in the intracellular and/or extracellular spaces of the brain. It can be caused by the body's response to a stroke. It most often occurs within 5 days of the stroke. It is more common in hemorrhagic strokes. This can become an emergency if not treated. The increase in fluid within the confined space of the skull can force the brain to herniate down into the spinal column compressing the brain and its vital blood flow.

Herniation
Signs of Herniation
- *Neuro changes*: ALWAYS call the doctor.
- *Decreased level of consciousness*
- *Pupil changes*
- *Abnormal breathing*: caused by impaired brain stem function
- *Decorticate posturing, abnormal flexion*: wrist and arms flexed, legs extended and rotated inward
- *Decerebrate posturing, abnormal extension*: arms extended with wrist rotated and flexed, legs extended and rotated inward
- *Cushing's triad*: a late sign of increased intracranial pressure; an increase in widening pulse pressure (difference between systolic and diastolic pressures), bradycardia, and abnormal respirations

Diagnosis
- STAT CT scan
- Intracranial pressure monitor (ICP): If the patient already has an ICP monitor, you can trend the patient's pressure and closely monitor for any changes. (See chapter 6, "Critical Care and Interventions" for more details on ICP monitoring.)

Cerebral Edema
Treatment for Cerebral Edema
- *Mannitol*: This osmotic diuretic is given IV. This will quickly pull fluid out of the cellular spaces of the brain, thereby reducing intracranial pressure.
- *Corticosteroids*: These IV steroids are given to suppress the body's immune response.
- *Surgical intervention*: A piece of the skull is removed to allow the brain to expand out of the skull instead of down into the spinal column. The piece of the skull may be stored in the patient's abdominal cavity or in the hospital's lab.

(See in chapter 7 Case Study 4 for a real-life example of a patient who suffered complications of cerebral edema.)

Hemorrhagic Conversion
So, we have learned that an ischemic stroke is a blockage of blood flow to a part of the brain. When this area is deprived of oxygen-rich blood for any period, the cells affected will die or become impaired.

Now the patient is in the hospital, and the medical team is trying every effort to intervene and reperfuse the ischemic area. However, this injured part of the brain may not be able to handle reperfusion or blood flowing through it. If this is the case, the blood vessels will leak blood into the brain.

This ischemic stroke has now converted to a hemorrhagic stroke. It is more common in patients who have received tPA. Maintaining the patients' blood pressure below 180/105 after receiving tPA can help reduce the risk of a hemorrhagic conversion.
(See in chapter 7 Case Study 3 for a real-life example of a patient who suffered a hemorrhagic conversion stroke.)

Seizures

A seizure happens when the electrical activity in the brain becomes chaotic resulting in repetitive abnormal muscle movements. Seizures usually last a few seconds to a few minutes. Patients may be unable to follow commands or appear to be looking in the distance while having a seizure. Seizures can be as simple as facial twitching or as serious as full-body convulsions. It is the nurse's job to maintain the patient's safety while she is having the seizure. The patient has no control over her movements.

Patients who have had strokes are more likely to have seizures; about 5% to 10% will have one or more seizures. The patient is more likely to have a seizure in the immediate days following her stroke. Seizures are more common in patients who have had a hemorrhagic stroke.

For a novice to patients with neurological problems, seizures can be very scary. You may turn your back for a second and all of the sudden the patient that was just talking to you is unresponsive and twitching. It's just you and your patient. What do you do? Call a code? Call the charge nurse? You feel helpless.

If Your Patient Starts to Seize
- Call for help. It's OK to yell, "I need help!" Or you can call the charge nurse or another coworker. If the patient is still breathing and has a pulse, there is no need to call a code.
- Place oxygen on the patient.
- Time the seizure and monitor the patient's body movements.
- Call the doctor to report seizure activity and request Ativan if not already available.
- Administer Ativan as soon as possible.

Nursing Interventions for Seizure Precautions
- Pad the side rails.
- Have oxygen ready.
- Have suction at the bedside.
- Keep the patient on bed rest if possible.
- Have an order of PRN Ativan.

Other Complications
The following is a list of a few additional complications commonly seen in stroke patients. Because most of these are not specific to stroke patients—but more specific to acute or chronically ill patients—we will not go into further details.

- Pneumonia
- Aspiration pneumonia
- Urinary tract infection
- Falls
- Deep vein thrombosis
- Pressure sores
- Contractures
- Shoulder pain

5
NURSING CARE AND CONSIDERATIONS

"Time is brain." You may have heard this saying before. It refers to the importance of quick treatment for the person having the stroke. As time goes by without treatment, brain cells are lost.

Here are some head-spinning statistics that will make you want to sprint when you are treating your stroke patient:

- Around 2 million neurons die for every minute that oxygen-rich blood is blocked from getting to brain cells. In a healthy person, it takes about 3 weeks for that many cells to die.
- The brain ages 3.6 years for every hour without treatment.
- Strokes are the 3rd-leading cause of death in the United States.
- Approximately 90% of strokes are ischemic. This means that there is a potential to treat these patients with the clot-busting drug tPA or perform other special procedures that can restore blood flow.
- Patients have around a 3-to-4.5-hour window to receive tPA from the moment that their symptoms start.

- Once the patient arrives in the emergency department, it can take up to 1 hour before the tPA is actually started.

Here are a few more startling statistics from the Centers for Disease Control and Prevention:
- Strokes are the leading cause of long-term disability.
- One in 4 strokes recur in someone who has already suffered a stroke.
- People with atrial fibrillation are 5 times more likely to have a stroke.
- High blood pressure is one of the most important modifiable risk factors.
- The death rates for strokes are higher in African Americans than in other groups.
- 75% of strokes occur in people over 65 years of age.

Impaired Communication

The medical team should consult speech therapy if the patient is having trouble with communication. Speech therapists are highly trained in working with stroke patients to help regain, relearn, or utilize strategies that will help the patient better communicate.

Types of Impaired Communication
- *Dysphagia*: may affect the patient's speech, ability to understand, and reading and writing skills (It doesn't affect the patient's intelligence.)
- *Receptive aphasia*: difficulty understanding what is being said
  - Speak slowly to patient.

- Use simple phrases.
- *Expressive aphasia*: difficulty speaking
  - The patient may speak slower or say the wrong word.
  - The patient can use picture boards.
  - Give the patient paper to write words.
- *Global aphasia*: difficulty understanding and speaking
- *Dysarthria*: difficulty speaking clearly because of weakness to the muscles that produce sounds
  - Use picture boards.
  - Write words.
- *Dyspraxia*: poor movement and coordination of the muscles to produce words; a communication disconnect between the brain and the muscles
  - The patient may repeat herself multiple times trying to get the right sound out.
  - Use picture boards.
  - Write words.

Swallow Precautions

Any patient admitted with a stroke should have a swallow screen completed. As mentioned earlier, you can do this with liquid, or you can wait for a speech therapist.

After a patient is made NPO by the nurse, a speech therapist will come to the patient's bedside and perform a detailed swallow evaluation. This can take up to 30 minutes. The speech therapist looks for weakness in the swallow muscles by trialing different food consistencies. Sometimes a modified barium swallow or fiberoptic endoscopic evaluation of swallowing (FEES) is ordered to get a more detailed look at the patient's swallow. Neither of these tests requires any action by the nurse. They are both minor with no preparation or risk involved.

As mentioned earlier, speech therapy will help guide the doctors and nurses on what type of diet is appropriate. The food options include regular, diced, ground, and pureed. The drink options include thin, honey thick, and nectar thick. You can use a thickener to make any beverage the appropriate consistency.

Some patients are not safe to swallow any food or liquid. These patients may have a small-bore feeding tube placed in their nose. They may be on a continuous feeding pump of liquid nutrition through their feeding tube. Consult your dietician to help the doctor determine the appropriate nutritional supplement the patient should receive.

Bowel and Bladder Issues

After a patient has had a stroke, he may become incontinent of his bowels and/or bladder. Offer your patient the option to go to the bathroom every 2 hours. If the patient is not fully conscious, turn, reposition, and check the brief every 2 hours.

Also, it is important to understand that your patient may not be able to communicate his needs and tell you that he needs to use the bathroom. If your patient becomes agitated or frustrated, make sure you offer the toilet.

Mobility

Patients who have had a stroke suffer from weakness. The location of the weakness depends on the location of the stroke.

> **Important Point**
> If the infarct happens on the right side of the brain, then the left side of the body will be weak and vice versa.

It is very important to enlist the physical and occupational therapy teams in the patient's multidisciplinary team. The therapist will work with the patient to regain some or all of her strength through exercises. Occupational therapy will assist the patient in the same manner but focus more on helping the patient to resume and/or modify her activities of daily living so that she may maintain her independence.

Fall Prevention

Stroke patients don't often realize the severity of their deficits and newfound weakness. They may try to get out of bed, not realizing that they can no longer stand. For this reason, it is very important to strictly follow all fall precautions.

Here are key fall prevention interventions to follow:
- Bed alarms (Make sure it is on and LOUD every time you walk out of your patient's room.)
- Chair alarms
- Lap belts for sitting up in the chair
- Fall socks
- Fall bracelets
- Fall signs

Pain Management

Managing pain in the initial period following a stroke can be tricky. Stroke patients may have very painful acute headaches, especially after a hemorrhagic stroke. You should always strive to relieve your patient's pain, but treat it carefully because sedating medications can mask or mimic worsening stroke symptoms. For this reason, some doctors order fentanyl for its short half-life. This is a heavy narcotic but typically wears off quickly. Always monitor your patient's response to fentanyl, and start with the lowest dose. If you don't have fentanyl available, then start with the mildest oral medication available.

If your patient's symptoms appear to be worsening, and you are questioning if the narcotics are impacting these changes, you may need to give Narcan to reverse the effects of the narcotics. Make sure you notify the doctor of what is going on before you proceed.

Emotional Support

As the nurse, remember that your patient has just been hit with a major life change. His life will never be the same. He doesn't even understand how much it will change yet. He may never go back to his home. He may never make it out of the hospital. Statistically, his mortality rate just went up. It is a huge amount for the patient and family to digest. Many of these patients were walking and talking and had normal lives before they came to the hospital.

Also, remember the family. Reassure them that it is OK to go home. Get their phone numbers, call them, and update them before you leave for the day. This is a long painful process for them too. They need rest just as much as the patient does.

It is your job to guide the patient and family through this process. Tell them what to expect each day and why you are doing the things that you do. You can find patient-friendly handouts on the Internet about diagnostic tests and medications. Family members are probably overloaded with information and from people telling them things, so write it down or print it out so they don't have to remember. By doing all of these things, you can tremendously reduce their anxiety.

Discharge Planning

It is important to include the case manager and social worker in the stroke patient's interdisciplinary care team. The patient will probably need to go somewhere before going home.

Options include the following:
- *Outpatient rehab*: The patient can go home and comes to therapy several times per week on an outpatient basis.
- *Rehabilitation hospital*: Inpatient rehab hospital where patients are required to do intensive therapy several times per day. Patients can still receive medications and are cared for by nurses.
- *Long-term acute care (LTAC)*: This type of facility is appropriate for patients who still need extensive care but aren't appropriate for the hospital (trach care, vent management, wound care, tube feeding).
- *Skilled nursing facility (SNF)*: This type of facility is appropriate for patients who may require more

45

care than a family can provide at home, care such as bathing, turning, and toileting.

- *Home health*: This is a service where an aide or nurse comes to the patient's home for help with various things.

The patient and family may need help from the case manager and social worker to arrange for assistive devices, such as a walker, wheelchair, bedside commode, shower chair, or oxygen.

It is a good idea to start talking with the family when the discharge is approaching about what they are comfortable with doing. Also, if they plan to take their family member home, then include them in your bedside care. They can assist with bathing, turning, and changing briefs. Sometimes after helping, some family members may realize that it is too much for them to handle at home.

6
CRITICAL CARE AND
INTERVENTIONS

Two important interventions are ventriculostomy (ventric) and external ventricular drain (EVD). You can consider both, quite literally, as brain drains.

Ventric and EVD

A tube is inserted into one of the ventricles in the brain to drain off cerebrospinal fluid (CSF). The neurosurgeon may insert this if the patient is showing signs of swelling. If you remove some of the fluid, there is room for the brain to expand, which will prevent herniation. Also, once the tube is in place, you can monitor the patient's intracranial pressure (ICP).

If you have never seen such a tube inserted, be prepared! The neurosurgeon literally hand drills into the patient's skull while you hold the patient's hand and comforts her. This is one of those times you will definitely think to yourself, "If my family and friends only knew what I do at work."

You will assist the neurosurgeon with the drain setup once the sterile procedure is completed. The drain will be connected to tubing and a bag, which will all be hung on an IV pole and leveled at the patient's tragus or external auditory canal. The surgeon will order the level that she wants the drain to be kept at.

Monitor the drain hourly for amount, color, and clarity. Notify the physician of any significant changes. If the patient sits up suddenly, this can cause overdrainage. You should close the drain stopcock for any repositioning, movement, or transport.

Change the drainage bag when it is 3/4 full. Make sure to wear sterile gloves and a mask, and use sterile technique any time you open this closed system. This is a direct open line to the inside of the brain. Infections are the most common complication.

Intracranial Pressure Monitoring

Normal ICP is 0–10 mmHg. Above 20 mmHg is an emergency! Zero the monitor and level your drain at least every 12 hours. Always assess for a good ICP waveform.

Cerebral Perfusion Pressure (CPP)
CPP = MAP (mean arterial pressure) − ICP (intracranial pressure)

An ideal CPP ranges from 60 to 100 mmHg. This number is used to help assure that the brain is getting adequate perfusion. Also, the doctor may want to attempt to manipulate the CPP by adjusting the patient's blood pressure to better control ICP.

Tissue Plasminogen Activator (tPA)

tPA is a clot-busting drug used to treat ischemic stroke patients when their last known well time is within 3 hours (up to 4.5 hours in some cases) of presenting to the emergency department. Once the patient has received the medication through the IV, her symptoms may disappear. This doesn't happen in all cases. But the patient might show a drastic reduction in her neuro deficits with some residual weakness.

tPA is typically given in the emergency department. The patient is then transferred to the ICU for close monitoring. In the first 24 hours after the tPA infusion, it is important to monitor the patient for bleeding and manage the patient's blood pressure. The blood pressure should be kept below 180/105. You should do neuro checks hourly during this time.

> **Caution: High-Risk Med**
> tPA is high-risk medication and not for everyone. There is a long list of contraindications that includes— but is not limited to—recent surgeries, recent stroke, head trauma, acute bleeding tendencies, severe uncontrolled hypertension, and history or current intracranial hemorrhage.

Intraarterial tPA

In cases when IV tPA isn't an option, the doctor may decide to give the tPA intraarterially. This procedure is done by a neuro interventionalist or interventional radiologist. The doctor will access the patient's femoral artery and guide a catheter up to the site of the blood clot in the brain. He then delivers a small dose of tPA at the site of the clot. This method poses a lesser risk of bleeding than IV tPA because the dose given is much smaller. This makes it ideal when patients don't qualify for IV tPA.

Craniotomy (Crani)

A neurosurgeon performs this type of surgery where the skull is opened for various reasons. Patients who undergo this type of surgery will require ICU care and monitoring postoperatively.

Aneurysm Clipping

Patients who have had a subarachnoid hemorrhage or have an unruptured aneurysm may undergo a craniotomy where the surgeon finds the bleed or aneurysm and uses a metal clip to cut off the blood supply to the neck of the aneurysm.

Think of the long skinny balloons that clowns use to make funny shapes at parties. Now think about how it would look if one of those balloons had a weak spot that bulged out like a cherry hanging. You don't want air to leak out of the weak spot, so you clamp it off, and the balloon is as good as new. This is similar to what happens when the doctor clips the aneurysm.

Craniectomy

When a patient has significant swelling in the brain, the doctor may have to remove part of the patient's skull to allow the swollen brain to expand. The removed piece of skull is stored in the hospital's laboratory and will be replaced in the patient once the patient recovers from the swelling. Postoperatively, the patient will require ICU care and monitoring.

Neurovascular Interventions

Cerebral Angiogram

Cerebral angiograms may be used for diagnostic purposes or as part of an intervention. This procedure is shorter and less invasive and requires less anesthesia than a craniotomy. The doctor inserts a catheter into the femoral artery and guides it up to the brain using x-ray imaging. Once the catheter reaches the brain, the doctor may perform an intervention or look at the brain's anatomy. The patient may or may not require ICU care postprocedure. If an intervention is performed, the patient will require closer monitoring. As with any procedure where the femoral artery is accessed, the patient must lay completely flat on bedrest for a number of hours to allow the artery to adequately clot off.

Stenting

While the patient is having his angiogram, the doctor may choose to place a stent in the vessel. This may be done because of narrowing or blockage in the vessel.

Coiling

Coiling is used to block off an aneurysm from within the vessel. The catheter delivers coils to the inside of the

51

aneurysm, which causes it to block off from circulation, making it impossible to rupture and cause a bleed.

7
CASE STUDIES

The following case studies are based on actual patients we have cared for. These are the most memorable patients for one reason or another. We take away from these stories 3 important points:

1. Chart well.
2. Perform thorough assessments.
3. Act fast when there are changes.

Case Study 1

R.H., a 72-year-old female, is brought to the emergency department by her husband after he came home from his morning walk to find her on the floor. R.H. has a history of high blood pressure and elevated cholesterol. She has difficulty speaking and right-sided weakness. Because her husband was away from the house when she fell, he is unable to tell the ED staff when she fell.

The neurologist examines her and notes that she has right-sided hemiparesis and global aphasia. She is awake and alert but nonverbal. She has right-sided facial droop, and opens eyes to voices. A CT scan is completed and shows a left middle cerebral artery infarct. Her NIH score on admission is 24.

Is R.H. a candidate for TPA? No. R.H. fell while alone, and her last time known well is unknown.

Plan of Care

- Permissive hypertension x 48 hours to help force blood to her brain tissue.
- Nursing swallow screen (She would automatically fail this because of her facial droop.)
- Continue any home antiplatelet or cholesterol medications.
- Start anticoagulant, if applicable, and proton pump inhibitor.
- Start intravenous antibiotics for possible aspiration.
- Telemetry.
- Echo.
- Repeat CT scan of brain in morning.
- Labs: TSH, B12, LFT, Lipids, HbA1C.
- Therapy: PT, OT, speech therapy.
- Possible rehab or skilled nursing facility.
- Patient and family education!

Case Study 2

D.W. is an active 65-year-old male. He rides his bike and swims laps in his pool 3 or 4 times per week. He has a history of high blood pressure and is taking an ACE inhibitor to manage it. Recently, D.W.'s ACE inhibitor dose was decreased because of a nagging cough he has been experiencing as a side effect. While in a meeting at work, D.W. had sudden difficulty speaking and fell to his left side when he tried standing up. His coworkers called EMS, and he was immediately taken to the hospital.

The neurologist examines him and notes that he has left-sided hemiparesis. He is awake and alert and has slightly slurred speech and a slight left facial droop. A CT scan is completed and shows a right middle cerebral artery infarct as a result of a 98% occluded right internal carotid artery. His NIH score on admission is 9.

Is D.W. a candidate for TPA? Yes. His last known well time was during his meeting, and his coworkers were able to report this to the first responders.

Plan of Care
- TPA administration followed by close neurological monitoring.
- Fall precautions.
- Nursing swallow screen (He would automatically fail this because of facial droop.)
- Restart blood pressure medications. Consider changing to beta-blocker.
- Start cholesterol medication to minimize risk of further buildup in vessels.
- Start anticoagulant, if applicable, and proton pump inhibitor.
- Start intravenous antibiotics for possible aspiration.
- Telemetry.
- Echo.
- Repeat CT scan of brain in morning.
- Labs: TSH, B12, LFT, Lipids, HbA1C.
- Plan for carotid endarterectomy.
- Therapy: PT, OT, speech therapy.
- Possible rehab or home health therapy.
- Patient and family education!

Case Study 3

B. H. was a 60-year-old male who was very active and healthy, other than his atrial fibrillation (AFib). He was admitted to the hospital for a special electrophysiology procedure to stop his AFib. The invasiveness of the surgery required his stopping the anticoagulants he was taking for AFib. The patient did well postoperatively and was transferred from the intensive care unit to the intermediate care unit on postop Day 1. He went back into AFib on postop Day 1. On postop Day 2, he remained in AFib but was feeling well.

He took a shower at 10 a.m. At 10:10 a.m., he called the nurse and asked her to put him back on telemetry. The nurse went in at 10:15 a.m. The patient was unable to speak; he had right-sided facial droop; and his right arm was weak.

The patient's head CT scan revealed an ischemic stroke. Because of the nature of his surgery, the neurologist decided that he was not a candidate for IV tPA despite being within the 3-hour window of treatment. An interventional radiologist was consulted and the patient was given intraarterial tPA.

The patient showed symptom improvement in the days following his procedure. His blood pressure was elevated, and he was requiring labetalol, hydralazine, and nicardipine. On the 3rd day after his intraarterial tPA, the patient showed significant worsening neuro status. His CT scan revealed a large hemorrhagic stroke in the area of his embolic stroke. He was not a candidate for any surgical intervention, and several days later he died.

Important Points

- B. H. was in AFib without being on anticoagulants.
- He was found almost immediately but was unable to receive IV tPA because of his surgery.
- He showed improvements with the intraarterial tPA.
- He had poor blood pressure control following his intervention, which led to his hemorrhagic stroke.

Case Study 4

S. M., a 36-year-old healthy female, presents to the hospital with the worst headache of her life and blurry vision. A CT scan reveals a ruptured AVM. She is admitted to the ICU after the neurosurgeon performs a coiling to her AVM. Her neuro checks remain unchanged with some improvement to her vision, so she is moved to a step-down unit the following day. She is still having headaches, which is to be expected given the size and location of her bleed.

In shift change report on postop Day 2, the night nurse reported giving the patient morphine for her headache. During the shift change assessment, the patient seemed lethargic but was able to perform an adequate neuro assessment. The night nurse reported the patient having been up some during the night because of poor pain control.

The day nurse continued to monitor the patient and perform hourly neuro checks. After several hours, the day nurse continued to notice the patient wasn't waking up any more than during shift change, and it was now 5 hours since her last morphine. She decided to administer a PRN dose of Narcan to see if S. M. would wake. After giving the Narcan, the patient remained lethargic. The nurse immediately notified the neurosurgeon who ordered a STAT head CT scan and transferred the patient back to the ICU.

The CT scan revealed significant swelling in the brain with a midline shift. A STAT dose of IV mannitol was given while the doctor decided whether to take the patient to the OR for a crani. The patient had significant diuresis with the mannitol and began to show mild improvement. The doctor decided to wait on surgery, given her improvement, but to monitor her closely and repeat another head CT scan later. The patient continued to improve and was discharged from the hospital later with no further interventions.

Important Points
- The night nurse should have given fentanyl instead of morphine.
- The nurses performed a shift change assessment.
- The nurse was vigilant by performing hourly assessments and called for changes.

CONCLUSION

Hello again,

We want to thank you for purchasing this book! We hope it was an easy-to-understand resource that will help you to better care for your patients.

If you enjoyed this book, then we would like to ask you for a favor. Would you be kind enough to leave a review for this book on Amazon? We would greatly appreciate it!

Don't forget to check us out on Facebook, Instagram (@nurse_ology), and Nurseology.com to see what other cool products we offer.

If there is a book topic you would like to see in the future, please email us at info@nurseology.com.

Thank you and good luck!

Jill and Kate

REFERENCES

American Stroke Association (2016). Types of Stroke. Retrieved from http://www.strokeassociation.org/STROKEORG/AboutStroke/TypesofStroke/Types-of-Stroke_UCM_308531_SubHomePage.jsp

American Stroke Association (2016). Stroke Risk Factors. Retrieved from http://www.strokeassociation.org/STROKEORG/AboutStroke/UnderstandingRisk/Understanding-Stroke-Risk_UCM_308539_SubHomePage.jsp

Centers for Disease Control and Prevention (2015). Stroke Facts. Retrieved from http://www.cdc.gov/stroke/facts.htm

Damodaran O, Rizk E, Rodriguez J, Lee G. (2014). Cranial nerve assessment: a concise guide to clinical examination. *Clinical Anatomy.* 27(1): 25–30. doi:10.1002/ca.22336

Gocan S, Fisher A. (2008). Neurological assessment by nurses using the National Institutes of Health Stroke Scale: implementation of best practice guidelines. *Canadian Journal of Neuroscience Nursing.* 30(3), 31–42.

Jauch EC, Saver JL, Adams HP, et al. (2013). Guidelines for the early management of patients with acute ischemic stroke: a guideline for healthcare professionals from the American Heart Association/American Stroke Association. *Stroke.* 44 (3): 870. doi: 10.1161/STR.0b013e318284056a

Printed in Great Britain
by Amazon

59152336R00036